# Wake Up Body:We Have Cancer

*by Daniel K Gartlan*

**Wake Up Body: We Have Cancer**

Copyright © 2014 by Daniel K Gartlan

# Table of Contents

# Why I Wrote This Book

When the number of people that are being diagnosed with Cancer and opting out of treatment continues to rise, then we need to take note. They are not opting out because of some "magic bullet cure". For the majority has no knowledge of any treatment except the conventional treatment of surgery, radiation and chemotherapy. It is the fear of these treatments and the eventual outcome that has cancer victims opting out. For it is historical knowledge from 60 plus years of these treatments that is fueling the new "opting out" option. We all have been touched by cancer through a loss of a family member, friend or loved one. We have all seen those brave and trusting souls fight to stay alive, just one more day but to no avail. It is this firsthand knowledge of the horrific pain, sickness and suffering that we have witnessed and has finally been cemented into our minds that allow us to face the reality that the "Trinity of Suffering" of conventional treatment is a failure. So opting out even with such a fatal disease is becoming more common. Opting out of known torturous treatment and eventual horrific death to a more dignified death with much less suffering and pain. We continue to be confined to the "legal" treatment of surgery, radiation and chemotherapy by a class of officials and government agencies that have complete power over our wellbeing and they are failing us. For people, with no knowledge of any other viable option, to refuse medical treatment shows just how we have lost faith in our medical system. That speaks volumes and needs to be addressed. A loss of faith due to a refusal to admit failure with a worldwide yearly cancer loss count of around 8.2 million is criminal and insane. We are losing an estimated 22,465 precious souls a day to a system of inferior and ineffective medicine. I pray that we Wake Up to this travesty and begin saving these precious men, women and children that are paying the ultimate price in the name of ego, money and power.

Such is the story of my mother who chose to let go of her fears and let her lung cancer consume her with no medical intervention. She chose to live at least 4 years without telling anyone of her cancer. Not even her husband of 62 years at the time of her passing. It was her wish and so it was until 4 days before her death. It was only then that my father and then her family and friends learned of her cancer and her wish to withhold that information from us. It was that day, which would be her final day "awake" that we began to learn and realize how strong a lady she truly was. Exactly why she chose to deal with her cancer that way we may never fully understand or know. What we do know is that she did not want to spend her last years disfigured and suffering horribly. She saw too many of her family and friends die horrible deaths after trusting in the cancer regimen recommended by their doctors. So many people who did not even have one "good" day in the last year of their lives. Not one single good day. Instead, each and every one of those last days were spent feeling sick and miserable. She did not want that and she chose to die without allowing herself to be destroyed inside and out in a methodical and costly way. I will forever admire that in my mother. Even though she had no idea what the end would be like without the normal cancer treatment she knew it had to be far better than with the treatment. The end came but it wasn't horrific and she was surrounded by family and loved ones and she went in a dignified and fairly peaceful manner. I thank God that she spared US, her family and friends, the emotional stress and anguish of seeing her die the horrific and unnatural death that cancer victims struggle through after all can be done with the surgeries, radiation and chemotherapy treatments. For theirs is a wasted body and soul. Hers was still a vibrant and living soul within her body. Sure, she was dying of a cancer that consumed her life, but it was nothing compared to what we all have seen in others after all is done that can be done and the ultimate damage has set in. I believe her fear of the cancer treatments and what it would do to her and to her family, friends and loved ones were what led her to do what she did. Or better yet, led her to not do what most others in her situation do. The absolute difference in her death as compared to those of my other family members and friends that chose the treatments is so astonishing that the dangers and damage of the "Trinity of Suffering" cannot be denied in my opinion. So it is my hope and prayer that those of you who read this book do so with an open mind and let yourselves be guided by the truth in you and not by fear and emotions.

For it is up to you to do what is right for you and you alone. If I can help but one person to face Cancer with confidence and true knowledge of what Cancer is and how they can become a whole and healthy person again without the poisons and suffering common to Cancer treatments today, then I have honored my Mother and Her Life. May God Bless You!

What now? Now that you have been given the news and your whole world is crashing around you, what should you do next? Are chemo and radiation really for you? Are there any other options for you?

I am here to tell you that yes, there are other options available! In fact, not only are there options available, many have been successful in bringing cancer ridden bodies back to an outstanding and astonishing healthy condition.

In this book I will lead you through the conventional allopathic view of treating cancer. I shall also lead you through some of the most amazing alternative and natural treatments that can bring a cancer stricken body back to a more natural state of being. Thus allowing your own body to be able to not only deal with the cancer but also eradicate the cancer in many instances. Please notice that I have stated that your body would be the healer; not any drugs, herbs or any other substance taken by you. For, all healing comes from within and from your own body. But, your body cannot and will not heal itself without being in a state of homeostasis. A few of the modalities that I shall put forth in this book might be little known by a majority of people. However, that does not mean that they should be overlooked or that they are any less successful than any of the others.

Through time there have been numerous successful and documented cancer treatments. These were successful in the treatment and in some instances eradication of the so called disease without using the highly toxic and deadly chemo and radiation treatments.

Let me be perfectly clear that I am not a medical doctor and I am not suggesting that you forgo any medical advice or treatments that you feel comfortable with. What I am suggesting is that you take control of your own body and health. You need to open your mind to the power that is innate within yourself. The treatment of cancer from the earliest days, until the present day, has changed very little. What has changed is the adding of specialized fields of diagnostics, treatments, so called research and surgery. This has created a labyrinth of confusion and a detachment of the medical field from any form of sensible and healthy views of the causes and treatments that could and would bring about healing.

Conventional Medical modalities attack tumors and cancer with external treatments that have changed very little in the many years of cancer recognition and treatment. The normal treatment options are surgery, radiation and chemotherapy of sorts. The patients are subjected to what amounts to criminal treatment. A torture of the sort that has been proven time and again to be mostly ineffective and many times bring about a more malignant condition within the body and will cause a more aggressive cancer condition.

All mainstream and allopathic medicine in this country puts forth an aura of fear and negativity where any cancer diagnosis is concerned! The populace of our country has been very successfully programmed into an intense and deadly fear of cancer and its treatment. This need not be so. All persons diagnosed with cancer should be told what needs to be done to get healthy and beat this so called disease.

So allow me to take you on an educational journey to bring about health and vitality instead of fear and hopelessness.

# Chapter 1-What Is Cancer?

The first thing you must attempt to understand should be; what is cancer? Is it an errant out of control cells growing uncontrollably and killing healthy cells? An action that is horribly destructive and extremely difficult to treat and attack? Something so complex that only highly trained medical specialists with the latest and greatest drugs and machines could possibly have any chance in dealing with?

Or, could it be a natural reaction of your body to protect itself from harm that you have done to yourself and from the toxins and abuse from our surroundings. Is it a natural reaction to protect life itself or a reaction and action emanating from the divine intelligence that resides in each and every cell of our being?

The earliest signs of cancer have been found on mummies from Peru and Egypt that date back to 3000 BC. The Edwin Smith Papyrus was originally written in 3000 BC and talked of tumors that were treated by cauterizations. This seems to be the oldest written description of Cancer.

Yet it was around 400 BC that Hippocrates first used the words "carcinos" and "carcinoma" to describe tumor growths. It was at that time that the word "cancer" was coined by Hippocrates being derived from the Greek word "karkinos" which means crab. It is believed that this was the phrase he used to describe the blood vessels on the tumors as they seemed to resemble the claws of a crab reaching outward. Hippocrates advised against any treatment as he said those people who did receive treatment of the cancers did not live long.

Throughout the years since Hippocrates, there have been many different views and theories put forth about the causes and correct treatment of cancer. During those years we discovered x-ray, radiation treatment and chemotherapeutic treatment. Of course we have not deviated from the earliest form of treatment noted on the mummies and kept up through the years and still today. I am referring to surgery for the removal of tumors. What we have done since the late 30's is kept up a regimen of surgery, radiation (radium) and chemotherapy with very little change.

So what does cause cancer? Once again the opinions and so called experiments lead to different conclusions. Some say cancer is caused by a virus while another camp believes it is caused by hormones and another by parasites. Of course, many more theories and conclusive testing's have pointed to an exuberant number of possible causes.

I guess any and/or all of the above and more could be part of the cancer problem, but I believe that if so, they are so only on a secondary cause level and not the Primary cause.

So what is the Primary cause of cancer? I am so glad you asked because in 1923 the primary cause was discovered. It was discovered through research being done at the Kaiser Wilhelm Institute by a brilliant medical doctor, physiologist and biochemist. His story is part of the story of cancer that has not been told. His research and subsequent discovery would and can impact the epidemic state of cancer that is present in society today. Impact it in a way only hoped for by the millions that are trying to survive cancer and even trying to survive the horrific cancer treatment that is the norm and pushed by every traditional doctor around. I shall tell you the story about his discovery and other treatments as well. Get ready to learn the truth behind cancer. It is not as complicated as you have been led to believe.

# Chapter 2-The Brilliance of Otto Warburg

Was the brilliance of Otto Warburg his earned accomplishments such as his Doctor of Chemistry degree or his degree of Doctor of Medicine or his biochemistry degree? Was it the fact that he was considered one of the 20th century's leading biochemists?

Was his brilliance in the fact that he was nominated an unprecedented 3 times for the Nobel Prize in Physiology or Medicine for three separate achievements? Was his brilliance in the fact that he won the Nobel Prize in Physiology or Medicine 2 times, once in 1931 and the second time in 1944 during the war? It was the second Nobel Prize that he was not allowed to accept as he was a Jew living in Germany during that time.

His brilliance was all of the above and even more. So much that Albert Einstein, a family friend, urged Otto to leave the army after WWI and return to academia so the world would not suffer the tragedy of the loss of his talent. His brilliance led to his being appointed as the Director of the Kaiser Wilhelm Institute for Cell Physiology. His brilliance was at a level that the German government created "The Otto Warburg Medal" to commemorate his outstanding achievements. It is regarded as the highest award for molecular biologists and biochemists in Germany.

Yet, all of these things and much more that he did and accomplished isn't the "brilliance" of Otto Warburg. The absolute brilliance of Otto Warburg was the work he did that discovered the **"Primary and real cause of Cancer"**. Let me state that again. His brilliance was his research and the end discovery of **THE PRIMARY AND REAL CAUSE OF CANCER**. It is this discovery that trumps all other accomplishments and feats that Otto Warburg reached during his amazing and brilliant life here on earth. His research led to his proven discovery of the primary cause of cancer. No other person had ever been able to isolate without exception the primary cause of cancerous cells. He did and for that was awarded the Nobel Prize in Physiology and Medicine. So who was Otto Warburg?

# Chapter 3-Otto Warburg A German Jew

Adolf Hitler brought mankind to the edge of insanity and destruction. Just the sound of his name conjures up thoughts of the evil that he gave life to during his control of the Nazi regime. His wholesale slaughter of 6 million Jews just because they were Jews is unprecedented in modern history. No other man in history has such a legacy of shame and destruction. No one was safe against the tyrannical madness of this man and his followers. Children, women and men of every race and nationality were targeted and murdered at the whim of Adolf Hitler. Jews especially, were murdered without any chance of being saved or spared under his rule. Even the slightest bit of Jewish bloodline would bring about retaliation and eventual death by horrible means. No Jew was to be spared in his "Final Solution" program.

On May 23, 1935 Adolf Hitler underwent surgery to remove a polyp on his larynx. Hitler was known to have an extreme fear of cancer. He believed he had stomach cancer due to an ongoing and constant problem with indigestion and flatulence. The growth of a polyp in his throat only made his fear of cancer increase and no assurance from his doctor could sway his belief nor ease his fears. He was positive he had throat cancer along with stomach cancer.

It was this fear that gave the world a gift that has been ignored, but is possibly the greatest discovery related to cancer. In fact, his fear of cancer enabled and allowed the ongoing research into the **PRIMARY CAUSE** of cancer and its reversal. It is this knowledge that has within its own information the cure for cancer. Sadly, the discovery has been ignored and no one or no entity within modern and traditional medicine has embraced the information to bring about a cure.

As the world was at war and Hitler and his government were methodically implementing his Final Solution to rid the world of Jews, there was one Jew that was seemingly protected. His name was Otto Heinrich Warburg and he was born of a Jewish father and a Christian mother. It was this pairing that should have sealed the fate of Otto Warburg who by that time was a distinguished physiologist, medical doctor and a biochemist that had already received a Nobel Prize in Physiology or Medicine in 1931 for his research and discovery in 1923 of the primary and real cause of cancer. During the Hitler Germany years, Otto Warburg continued his research into cancer and it was during these years that he was able to reverse the cancerous state of cells back into normal and healthy cells.

What was this great discovery that Otto made that earned him the Nobel Prize? He stated that his research proved that there are many secondary causes of cancer, but that there is only one Primary and real cause of cancer. This primary cause of cancer is oxygen deficiency brought about by toxicity and other secondary conditions in the body. His research demonstrated that all forms of cancer have two basic conditions present. These two conditions are a lack of oxygen at the cellular level (hypoxia) and acidosis.

What Otto Warburg discovered was that he could deprive a cell of 35% of its oxygen needs and within 48 hours it could turn cancerous. Otto Warburg said the following; *"Cancer, above all other diseases, has countless secondary causes. But, even for cancer, there is only one prime cause. Summarized in a few words, the prime cause of cancer is the replacement of the respiration of oxygen in normal body cells by a fermentation of sugar. All normal body cells meet their energy needs by respiration of oxygen, whereas cancer cells meet their energy needs in great part by fermentation. All normal body cells are thus obligate aerobes, whereas all cancer cells are partial anaerobes. From the standpoint of the physics and chemistry of life this difference between normal and cancer cells is so great that one can scarcely picture a greater difference. Oxygen gas, the donor of energy in plants and animals is dethroned in the cancer cells and replaced by an energy yielding reaction of the lowest living forms, namely, a fermentation of glucose. "*

Simply put, healthy cells will remain healthy as long as they are in an alkaline condition with proper oxygen supply to support cellular respiration whereas cancerous cells must have an environment of acidosis (acidic) and no oxygen. Once in a cancerous state of fermentation the cancerous cells must have sugar to feed upon. This obviously makes sugar a very important player within the Cancer Game. Unfortunately, the normal diet of modern day America and in fact most of the world contains an uninterrupted supply of said needed sugar from many sources. Another big problem is that a healthy diet needs to be at least 80% alkaline and 20% acidic. The majority of us has reversed this and ingest very little amounts of alkaline foods and way too much acidic or acid producing foods. This sets us up to be highly acidic by doing so and in that we are creating the environment of acidosis also needed to support cancer. Diet and nutrition is extremely important in dealing with cancer and/or preventing cancer. Otto found that without exception if a cell is in an alkaline state and is in a state of healthy respiration it will not become cancerous and without exception if a condition and environment of acidosis (too acidic) and a lack of oxygen is present the cell will change to a cancerous state. This obviously is a very simple generalization, but his research has pinpointed the cause that has been ignored.

His later research, which was done under the auspices of the Nazi regime, brought about amazing results in bringing cancer cells back to a healthy state. He found that by adding back a higher concentration of oxygen and bringing the cell pH level to an alkaline state that the cell could be brought back to a precancerous or noncancerous state. For this he was awarded a second Nobel Prize in Physiology and Medicine. Being a Jew in Germany under Hitler's rule, he was not allowed to accept the award. This is very ironic in that Adolf Hitler seemed to protect him from the treatment and "Final Solution" that all other Jews were being subjected to. He was known to be Hitler's authority on cancer and undoubtedly was protected by Hitler. . It seems that Hitler's fear of cancer and his knowledge of Warburg's research and discoveries may have spared Otto from arrest and even death. During the year 1941, because of his Jewish bloodline, he was removed from his position and research by the Nazi hierarchy. Within a few weeks he was reinstated to resume work on his cancer research per a personal order from Hitler's Chancellery.

What does his research and discoveries mean? It means that there are ways to help your body cure cancer. It is up to you to research and become the one who takes control of your own health and healing. If the conventional way is your choice, then by all means go that route. But, if you would like to go a more alternative route that considers this discovery which has been ignored then do your research. Get your eating habits to a healthier, more alkaline diet. Go to a Naturopathic doctor or talk to your doctor about alternative treatments.

Knowledge is everything when it comes to your health, healing and life itself. A must read book full of information from medical doctors that are using all natural and alternative methods in curing cancer is *"Knockout"* by Suzanne Somers. This book also addresses having conventional treatment along with alternative methods. So you can still do the radiation and chemo, but have other information to supplement that protocol. You can also find excellent articles online about using Ph treatments and oxygen treatments. An awesome site for pH information is www.phkillscancer.com. You can find informative articles about pH and cancer and oxygen treatments by searching them on www.naturalnews.com.

Research, research, research. That is what I can and will stress here. In the words of Dr. Warburg…. *"But nobody today can say that one does not know what cancer and its prime cause is. On the contrary, there is no disease whose prime cause is better known, so that today ignorance is no longer an excuse that one cannot do more about prevention. That the prevention of cancer will come there is no doubt, for man wishes to survive. But how long prevention will be avoided depends on how long the prophets of agnosticism will succeed in inhibiting the application of scientific knowledge in the cancer field. In the meantime, millions of men must die of cancer unnecessarily."*

# Chapter 4-The Trinity of Suffering

**C-A-N-C-E-R.** A six letter word that has grown to be one of the most dreaded words anyone would ever want to hear. A word that spreads fear and dread in the hearts and lives of those diagnosed with it and also their family, friends and loved ones that will also be affected. Before the "ordeal" is over, great damage will be done in the form of eventual death and even for the survivor's there will be damage in a form of mental, emotional and physical pain and suffering. Why does this have to be? Is it such a cruel and unrelenting disease that the only path during the struggle to survive is full of pain and suffering?

Cancer is the 'by-product', if you will, of a dis-eased and unhealthy body. It is a symptom so important that I consider it your body's last call for you to correct your lifestyle and get your magnificent body back into a healthy state of balance and back to a state of health so that it can go about healing itself of the causes of Cancer. I know many, many, many people will read this and say I am crazy or just a little off balance. But, I beg to differ with them. My words will give my point of view of this extremely deadly and profitable business of Cancer.

First of all it is hard for me to fathom how you can cure ANYBODY of ANY so called disease by radiating and poisoning/burning them. Let's say I go for a yearly medical exam. I pass with flying colors and am told I am as healthy as a horse. But, we want to give you chemotherapy and radiation treatments just because. Well, now, I in my blind, follow the advice, programmed stupor, feel so privileged to be chosen for such an honor, I say let's do it. So the very highly trained Cancer professionals with their very highly protected procedures begin this journey of radiation and chemo on me. Wow, what a shock to my once healthy immune system. After the first round of treatments I am a beaten man. But, I persevere under the doctor's advice and encouragement. My immune system, which is my body's healing system, has been overwhelmed and pretty much made useless. Now I am helpless in keeping my once healthy body strong and protected as I now have a highly compromised and weakened immune system. I feel miserable all the time and my quality of life has slipped to 'horrible'. Now I get the word that the Cancer has come back with a vengeance and is spreading rapidly. But WHOA now, I didn't even have Cancer before I started these procedures. Oh, that's right. Both the radiation and chemotherapy are known carcinogens. They, in and of themselves, can cause Cancer. Oh my word, why do they give it to people then???? Hmm....

Let's be honest here folks. The normal Cancer treatment protocol in the United States and most of the world at this time is; surgery, burn and poison. What I call the "Trinity of Suffering". The same it has been for 60 plus years. The treatment the medical field is offering to an already weakened person with an overtaxed immune system is to cut, burn and poison. What a marvelously intelligent way to proceed. I know that these recommendations come from some of the most brilliant minds in science and medicine and THAT my friend is the problem. They are stuck in their programmed box of schooling. Schooling and training that has been financed and written by men and women of a very narrow way of thinking and a very wide way of being profitable above all else. We are constantly inundated with a type of visual brainwashing that leads us to follow the advice of men and women who know little or nothing about us. We follow them into a Hell of cancer torture and debilitating treatments all with their knowledge that it really isn't that successful or healthy for any of the recipients of these called Cancer Treatments. They become our 'diseases' and our killers all in the name of "Medicine". Those that are the lucky survivors survive in spite of the chemo and radiation. They were the ones that were strong from the offset. They became the lucky ones that had a supreme support system in place and a very positive attitude. A positive attitude that had their eye on the prize of beating this awful scourge.

Just how bad is chemotherapy and what are the results? In an article By Dr. James Howenstine, MD. he wrote; *"What are results of chemotherapy drugs? Associate Professor Graeme Morgan of Australia was the lead researcher on an article titled "The contribution of cytotoxic chemotherapy to 5 year survival n adult malignancies." This research showed that chemotherapy improved 5 year survival by less than 3% in adults with cancer. In 1987 Dr. Lana Levi of the University of California wrote "most cancer patients in this country die of chemotherapy. It does not eliminate breast, colon, or lung cancer. This fact has been known for over a decade. Women with breast cancer are likely to die faster with chemotherapy than without it."*

Let's say you have Cancer. You give over your Life to "experts" that believe when all they can do fails, and it does very frequently, then it's time to look to God to save you. After they have taken a body that had a dis-ease and then totally destroy all chances of it to heal, then and only then do they admit defeat. But wait a minute. Which one in this horrible journey is really the defeated one? Which one of you will not live to see another day or another Christmas or another child or grandchild born? Who has given all they had in this medical adventure and has come up short? Chances are it is you. You the ever trusting patient is the one that has lost. All of this loss and insanity in the name of "Expert

Cancer Treatment" by "Experts in their field" have brought about this very sad ending. In most cases, simply because they do not believe and may not even allow the patient to try alternative treatments either as the primary or as a supplemental protocol. They have no faith in alternative treatments, and often times ridicule them and pronounce them as dangerous.

This declaration coming from someone that has no qualms about pumping you full of chemo and radiating you over and over and that has never studied herbs (the original medicine) or nutrition seems kind of ridiculous to me. It is time we believe in ourselves and make our own choices in this life or death situation. Don't go blindly into something with someone you don't know and who doesn't know you. You know yourself, so get all the information and ask questions and get more than one opinion. After all, whose job is it to cure Cancer? You or the doctor? It is up to you to take charge of your precious gift of life and correct what needs correcting to continue to thrive and live and Love!

Is chemo successful in treating cancers? Obviously not. In fact, in 1992 the German government published a report on the effectiveness of chemotherapy against cancers. The research and subsequent report found that there was no benefit in chemotherapy treatment except for childhood leukemia, some lymphoma, testicular cancer and Hodgkin's disease. In 2001 they published an updated report that confirmed the earlier findings that for most cancers chemotherapy does nothing. Yet, cancer patients are being subjected to the chemo and the damage done by the chemo.

Once again from the writings and research of James Howenstine, MD. *; The package inserts for chemotherapy drugs admit that taking a course of chemotherapy drugs can increase your risk of subsequently developing a new*

14

*cancer by about 10%. The National Institute for Occupational Safety and Health (NIOSH) warns that the powerful drugs used in chemotherapy can cause cancer in employees who handle them (nurses, pharmacists, cleaning personnel). If continued too long these drugs are fatal. The damage to white blood cells, killer lymphocyte and red blood cell production makes the patient vulnerable to overwhelming infection, which is the cause of death in many patients on chemotherapy and radiation. It never made sense to me why administering toxic substances that cause major side effects could possibly heal a serious illness like a malignancy.*

Dr. William Campbell Douglass II, MD stated *"To understand the utter hypocrisy of chemotherapy, consider the following: The McGill Cancer Center in Canada, one of the largest and most prestigious cancer treatment centers in the world, did a study of oncologists to determine how they would respond to a diagnosis of cancer. On the confidential questionnaire, 58 out of 64 doctors said that all chemotherapy programs were unacceptable to them and their family."* Now, that my friends, is total HYPOCRISY!

Chemotherapy drugs are so ineffective because they are administered without testing to see which would perform better. They are administered at the whim of the oncologist in many cases. You may very well be given whatever the "drug of choice" or "drug of the month" might be at the particular time of your treatments. Yet, the medical establishment along with the pharmaceutical industry knows and has known for decades that certain cancers and certain individual conditions negate any effects of chemotherapy.

So what is the right course? Chemotherapy drugs should not be used as you would a wide spectrum antibiotic. In fact, just like the testing that is done to pinpoint the best antibiotic for each job needed in bacterial infections, there is also a chemosensitivity test available. This test will help pinpoint which chemotherapy drug would have the best overall result in your treatment. But, it costs and it would require individual testing, which would "hold up" the efficient "one size fits all" in and out process of profitable impersonal cancer treatment.

I am going to mention two fairly recent studies done. I want you to realize that there have been many more than just these two so I would recommend you research for more studies. They are out there and in many cases are done by reputable Cancer Hospitals and Cancer Research Centers. I just want to make you aware that studies are being done and they are proving what many medical professionals have known for years. The media unfortunately rarely bring the results to the forefront of information access.

In a report released in February of 2014, researchers at UCLA's Jonsson Comprehensive Cancer Center, Department of Oncology discovered that, even though half of all cancer tumor cells were killed per radiation treatment, the radiation treatment itself on breast cancer actually transforms other cancer cells into cancer stem cells. Cancer stem cells have an extremely higher resistance to further treatment than do normal cancer cells. They simply found that radiation treatment for breast cancer (the choice of research) creates cancer and one that is more resistant to curing.

Another report was released in 2012 by the Fred Hutchinson Cancer Research Center in Seattle concerning chemotherapy. The Fred Hutchinson Cancer Research Center was established in 1975 and is considered one of the world's leading research centers. It was at the FHRC that bone marrow transplants were pioneered for leukemia and other blood related diseases. They discovered and documented that chemotherapy caused damage to healthy cells. The subsequent reaction of the once healthy cells is a secretion of a protein which is then used by the cancerous cells and accelerates the growth of the cancer cells. Not only causing an acceleration, but according to Peter Nelson of the Fred Hutchinson Cancer Center, who is the co-author of the study, once the protein is captured by the nearby cancer cells, it causes them to *"grow, invade, and importantly, resist subsequent therapy."*

As far as surgery for cancer tumor removal....well that too is causing problems and in many instances spreads the cancer through the blood stream and lymph system. A cancer tumor releases cancer cells into the blood stream. Some of those cancer cells will find another location to call home, but will not become active but remain dormant. It was through research from Judah Folkman that found that cancer tumors attract blood vessels to keep nourished and survive. This is known as **angiogenesis**. It was from this field of study and a presentation attended by Nöel Bouck by Judah Folkman that led to an amazing discovery and realization. Normal cells will secrete angiogenic inhibitors to inhibit new blood vessel growth. Once the cell becomes cancerous, they began producing blood vessel stimulators yet they still secrete inhibitors at a lower level than before. Once a tumor is formed, the tumor will release upwards of a million cancer cells into the bloodstream daily. Many of these do find a new "home" to locate to but may not become active at that time. In many instances they will remain dormant until the original tumor is removed. With the removal of the tumor, Nöel Bouck found that the inhibitor was also removed, allowing the other dormant cells to become highly active and aggressive. So as far as debating whether surgery causes spreading or not....well it seems in some cases the answer is yes.

# Chapter 5-The Angel Nurse and God's Healing Tools

Let me tell you about someone I consider an expert on Cancer Treatment. She had a very successful 50 plus year record of healing cancer in thousands of patients over that time period. Rene Caisse was a Canadian nurse who was given a recipe formula of herbs from a lady that had gotten the formula from an Ojibwa Indian healer to be used in treating cancers. The remarkable thing about this was that she made and administered this mixture for over 50 years to those in need. The very same patients that had been victimized by the conventional treatments of the normal cancer treatments of surgery, radiation (radium) and chemotherapy. The people that came to her had been given up on by their cancer doctors and allowed to see her as a last resort. Once their doctors had "done all we can do for you" they were allowed to seek out this wonderful Healing Angel. These were cases that were well documented with all necessary tests and documentation from the original doctors. It was only after these same doctors said there was nothing else to be done, did they allow their patients to go to Ms. Caisse for her treatments. They could be treated by her, but were to go back to their original doctors for follow up visits. It was then that it became very apparent to all these many doctors that these terminal cases were getting healed and in many instances starting to thrive again. Even in the cases where death did eventually come from the cancer, there was a great improvement and they noted that in many of those cases, they lived a lot longer than initially anticipated and without pain or very low amounts of pain. She was so successful in her treatments and healing that she came to the attention of the Canadian Government. It was through this "alignment", if you will, that she was supervised and all her work was highly documented by medical experts and Canadian Government medical experts. She was not allowed to administer her treatment without a written diagnosis of cancer from a medical doctor. Her treatment became the most successful and most documented treatment available. Her treatment became so successful that the Canadian Parliament came within 3 votes of declaring it a cure for cancer before the then equivalent of our AMA and pharmaceutical lobby put pressure on the members and high ranking officials to have it blocked as a cure. It was just too natural and readily available and too cheap.

This was an amazing woman who dedicated her life to healing others and only took donations when offered. Her life and journey of healing and her research under lab conditions with supervision by the government and medical professionals are all well documented and written about. A very good and informative book is "Calling of An Angel" written in 1988 by Dr. Gary Glum. Rene Caisse called her formula "Essiac" as in her last name in reverse. It is also called 4 Herb Tea. The 4 Herb tea formula and also the herbs to make Essiac are available through a few sources. One of the most reliable suppliers with the highest quality herbs and the 4 Herb Tea is Herbal Healer Academy at www.herbalhealer.com. On this site there are wonderful testaments from users about Essiac and 4 Herb Tea. I have been using 4 Herb Tea for years and it has also been noted to have many other medicinal uses. As with Dr. Glums' own experience, he used it to heal his chronic bronchitis. Take control and research for your own health and, in cancer situations, your life! As I always state in my blogs; do something at least. Just don't leave it up to someone else.

I am passionate when it comes to the poor innocent men, women and children being killed by our typical medical treatments. Millions are dying needlessly because of greed and power and ego. That this country and world have come to that is totally abhorrent and opposite of the Hippocratic Oath. We ALL deserve a life of health and wellbeing. Please, please if you have cancer or know someone who has cancer, take the time to research this amazing gift of nature that can help your amazing body heal itself. It can even be taken with chemo and radiation, but I personally would not do that. In fact, I would bring about my healing naturally with a more natural and alkaline diet along with Essiac.

The writings contained in this book are strictly my thoughts, concerns and opinions being expressed as my Right to free speech. I am in no way advising anyone not to seek professional medical help but I am putting forth my opinion that we do have the right to treat ourselves as we see fit whatever that may mean to you the reader. I do not agree with medical treatments as such and believe the treatments are causing the deaths of countless thousands of people in a reckless and needless and horrible manner. But, once again, that is my opinion as stated here. My only hope here is that this article may spur someone into taking control of their own life and healing. I write these words, hoping that people will seek out more information about this wonderful natural healing recipe and that through the information and herbs people will live!

# Chapter 6-Otto's Discovery and the Alkaline, pH Way

As part of the ongoing research and experiments that Otto Warburg performed, he discovered that an alkaline condition supported healthy cellular respiration. He discovered that cancer cannot and will not survive under proper alkaline conditions. This is why it is so very important that we have a diet that creates that alkaline condition in our Holy Temples. The one and only vessel that we will have to reside in., Not only that, but also that we detoxify our bodies as needed from the toxicity that builds inside of us from our so called food and the environment.

The first line of defense in keeping the blood pH at the optimal range of 7.35-7.45, is through your diet. Vegetables and fruits should be the majority of our daily diet. Also, water is a life giving source that is often ignored or not taken seriously. So many of us are dehydrated and have no idea. We should be drinking well filtered and alkaline water if possible. It is so important to keep your cells hydrated properly plus water intake will help in counteracting acidic conditions. There are many excellent alkaline water machines available and you should research them. You can also make alkaline water by using the juice from ½ a lemon for every 6-8 oz. of water. Just add to filtered or spring water if available and let sit a few minutes and drink.

Beyond that, what can we do when we have been diagnosed with cancer to bring our body to an alkaline condition wherein cancer may not exist or where cancer will have to fight to exist? Believe it or not there are many natural ways to help your body to get the pH level back to an alkaline condition. Like I mentioned earlier, diet and water can be utilized. There are super greens that can also help. Spirulina, wheat grass and chlorella are just a few. Also, many people do the daily regimen of juicing greens that supercharge the ability of the body to absorb the nutrition and all the goods they have to offer you in your healing. I personally take spirulina and also Moringa Leaf powder which is an amazing plant nicknamed the "miracle tree". Take time to research this awesome gift of God that grows freely. This amazing Moringa plant has the following attributes and many more I will not list. But, according to Dr. Monica Marcu, who is a scientist and a pharmacologist, *"Moringa is a plant possessing an impressive nutrient profile and numerous therapeutic qualities. For instance, the plant contains hundreds of phytochemicals (plant-specific substances), nutritional compounds ranging from vitamins and minerals to omega fats and all essential amino acids. We also know it can clean and disinfect water (functioning even better than aluminum sulfate, a standard water flocculant), has antibacterial and antiviral properties, and contains powerful antioxidant and anticancer substances and other important compounds such as cytokinins (Zeatin). It also can function as a natural growth stimulant for other plants. Moringa has uses outside of the human health and medicinal realms - it is a terrific high nutrient feed for animals, it is useful in agro-forestry, and its oil has the potential to be used as biodiesel fuel. In many ways, Moringa truly appears to be a "miracle" plant."*

By far the one thing that I personally would do to bring about healing from cancer is what I call "the baking soda protocol". In fact, I do this as a preventive from time to time. It is so powerful and yet so simple just as our creator intended health to be. Now I know many have heard that mixing baking soda in a glass of water is good for different situations. Maybe your grandmother talked about it. Either way it works in bringing about a more alkaline state. And remember, Cancer doesn't do well in an alkaline condition. Let me turn you on to just one person among many that have used this procedure or something similar to become healthy again and according to them and their oncologists….Cancer free.

I would like to tell you about Vernon "Vito" Johnston. Vernon was diagnosed with class IV Aggressive Prostate cancer that had already spread to the bones. A suggestion from his son that he should find out more about pH as it affects the body led him to start his own research that within days had him starting a program of mixing baking soda, water and molasses to attempt to raise his pH level. By the time he started the program he had 10 days to take the baking soda before he was to be tested again. After sticking to his daily regimen of slowly increasing the amount of baking soda and the frequency of taking the drink he was able to bring his pH up to a higher alkaline level. After 10 days he stopped to have another bone scan. When the results of the bone scan arrived it stated, *"NO CONVINCING EVIDENCE OF AN OSSEOUS METASTATIC PROCESS"*. A few days later he received the news that his blood tests showed a PSA of 0.1! His original PSA was 22.3 and that is what raised the red flag in the beginning and started what he terms his "Dance with Cancer".

Vernon is only one of many documented cases where baking soda has been used successfully in treating cancer. He has and did progress into many more procedures in conjunction with the baking soda. He uses meditation, visualization, breathing techniques and definitive diet changes to bring about a more alkaline diet. He has a website with more information at www.phkillscancer.com and has written an extremely informative book about his story and how to adjust the baking soda program to better suit you. His book is titled

**"Vernon's Dance With Cancer....After the Jolt"** and a link is found on his website to order the book.

I must also mention Dr. Mark Sircus who is one of the leading doctors treating cancer with sodium bicarbonate. He is well respected in the medical community and has written a book; **"Sodium Bicarbonate: Rich Man's Poor Man's Cancer Treatment"**. His website can be found at http://drsircus.com/ and he can be contacted from that site for consultations.

There is more and more research on the efficacy of sodium bicarbonate in healing cancer. All of this leads back to part of Otto Warburg's discovery. That cancer cannot survive in an environment of alkalinity and oxygenation. I look forward to a day when people are being healed naturally without the horrible poisons and toxic materials that are the mainstay of allopathic cancer treatment now.

# Chapter 7-Detox, Detox, Detox

In today's environment we are constantly bombarded with toxins. Add to that our horrible diet and unhealthy habits and all of the toxic medicine that is so widely accepted and used and we become a time bomb of dis-ease waiting to go off. That is why it is imperative that you detox or remove the toxins from your body so your body can have a better chance of operating as it was intended to. It was created to heal itself in most instances, but only if it is in a proper state of balance.

People with cancer have a highly compromised liver and in most cases their kidneys are also compromised. When you have two of the most important filters of your body and blood overtaxed and toxic to the point of being ineffective, then you have a serious problem. One that probably has been a contributing factor in your health condition. Once these are too toxic and ineffective to do their jobs, then the results will touch every other organ of your body. It starts a domino effect in your body. Your problem becomes systemic and if you add surgery and radiation and chemotherapy drugs to the mix then you have a deadly cocktail with fatal possibilities. That is why it is imperative to detox.

If you research ways to detox you will find countless numbers of ways available to you. But, just like all things, there are good and there are exceptional and there are downright scams. You have to be diligent in this matter and find proven ways. I will tell you from personal experience that you should use gentle but effective detox protocols. Believe me they are out there and they do work.

I have tried many through the years to differing degrees of cleansing and to differing systems and whole body cleanses. I will say that Andreas Moritz is very knowledgeable about detoxing the liver and about cancer in general. His knowledge and detoxing help are very much appreciated and I love his writings about health.

Hands down the best tried and proven detox I have found is a full body detox from www.dherbs.com. All of his products are plant based organic and his products are the best. He has amazing knowledge available to anyone who will go to his site and search his site and the articles there.

So what is this Full Body Detox I am speaking of? It is a 20 day all natural, easy to follow program to detox and cleanse your body that will help purify and strengthen your body, including your immune system and excretory system. Your immune system will be enhanced by the 20 day cleanse which will allow your body to be more able to naturally bring about a stronger healing capability. You will receive complete information on how to perform the Cleanse for optimum benefit and results. As part of the program you will be advised to have a more alkaline diet of mostly vegetables and fruit. You will need to drop all sugars, red meats, wheat products and milk products from your diet. These are all acid producing and as such are detrimental to you reaching the healthy alkaline state you will need in your healing. All of this information is sent along with the cleanse kit or is readily available to you online at their website.

 Like I already stated, this is a simple but extremely effective and powerful natural tool for bringing healthier conditions for yourself no matter what dis-ease you may be dealing with. Is it difficult at all? What is difficult is breaking away from your bad habits of a very bad diet. That is why we may think it is difficult. Yet, like the website at Dherbs says; "if you can remove those unhealthy foods and habits from your life and diet for 5 days, then you can do 20 days!" Realize this people...this is a **MERE** 20 days we are speaking of. What a way to get on track to better health and begin a process of healing!

There are other all natural supplements and herbs that have an alkalizing affect and /or a cleansing ability. Many of the "Super Foods" are truly amazing in supplying our bodies with much needed nutrients and such. One such amazing plant that I mentioned earlier and that I take daily is the Moringa Oleifera powder. The Moringa benefits are too numerous to mention but it is known among many names as **"the miracle tree"** because of its many benefits and medicinal abilities. It has been proven in scientific and medical research to be one of the best plants for treating malnourishment as it contains around 40 antioxidants and over 90 nutrients. Just a few of the benefits that Moringa supplies; 25X more iron than spinach, 4X more protein than eggs, .75X more Vitamin C than oranges, 10X more Vitamin A than carrots, 15X more potassium than bananas and 17X more calcium than milk. On top of that it has many medicinal properties. This amazing plant is just becoming known here in the United States, but has been used and well known for years in other parts of the world. Remember the name for you will be hearing more and more about it. An excellent site for more info about this natural wonder is www.miracletrees.org and where I get my Moringa products from, www.ilovemoringa.com. Moringa plants are very hardy in a warm climate and can easily be planted and raised on your own, thus supplying you with your own renewable supply of health.

Let's not forget Spirulina and Chlorella. Both of these are food for your body and are all usable and healthy plants and herbs. These two are food at the cellular level of life. I also take Spirulina most days and sometimes Chlorella with the Spirulina. Both are algae. Chlorella is a single-cell green algae and Spirulina is a blue-green algae. Spirulina is one of nature's best suppliers of B12. In fact, it has the highest amount of B12 than any other known natural source. You should research these two staples for maintaining your health also.

Making a shift to a more raw diet is critical in allowing your body to de-stress and rid itself of toxins and parasites. Once again, you can find hundreds of awesome recipes for a raw and/ or vegetarian type diet. Going to that type of diet does not have to be boring. In fact, many people find that after they "dump the junk" from their diets long enough for their bodies to adjust to the healthier foods, that they lose the desire for junk and sugar. They have been known to feel nauseous after ingesting junk food afterwards. This is the inherent divine intelligence of your body letting you know that you are harming your body with junk and toxic foods. Take heed when that happens and get back into a proper and healthy diet.

# Chapter 8-My Preferred Plan of Healing

What is my preferred plan to heal from Cancer? Quite simply, it is just as I have written about. First, I should have no fear of Cancer. I should have complete faith in my ability to heal. This ability is within each and every one of us and is much stronger than any cancerous condition. But, we must prepare, allow and give our body what it needs to eradicate Cancer. We do that with cleansing our body, mind and spirit. We do that with proper herbs and plants to bring about a detoxing. And we meditate or do relaxation exercises. We nourish our body, mind and spirit with proper diet and amazing God given plants and herbs and super foods. We alkalize through natural means and a more raw or vegetarian diet. We laugh often and seek positivity in each and every day.

Finally, we begin one of over 200 proven all natural Cancer cures available to us. Many of these seem to be very hard to find out about without a lot of research. So you must research for your Life. Many of these are historically proven, but are being called quackery by those that really know nothing about them yet fear for their livelihoods because of the affordability of these cures. I have listed only a few, but many other programs are out there and more and more doctors are starting to find amazing results naturally and are beginning to talk about it. Keep yourself educated and informed. Just one protocol that has great promise, but it is hitting roadblocks at this time is *Cannabis Oil.* This is an absolute awesome tool for Cancer healing that I know will eventually be made available. In America, Cancer is now the leading cause of death in children between the ages of 1 and 14. And the leading cause of death in adults. According to

US National Cancer Institute, there is a ***new cancer diagnosed in America every 30 seconds***. An estimated one person dies of Cancer in just the U.S. alone every minute. This because we have an unearned blind trust in others. We believe they are the only ones that know what is best for us. This because we allow a course of treatment that is known to be an overall failure. This because we do not take the time to be our own advocate in saving ourselves. These numbers are horrific and are lost lives that could have been saved in many instances with proper help and knowledge. ***WE MUST DO BETTER AS A COUNTRY AND AS A WORLD IN SAVING OUR PRECIOUS FELLOW HUMAN BEINGS.*** I hurt inside knowing that so many beautiful people are suffering and being maimed to no avail. My hope is that someone will read my book and begin their own decision making and research that will save their life or someone they know and that that person will spread the word and a domino effect of choosing to live and heal from cancer will explode onto the world scene. We all deserve a happy, healthy life and health care that does not harm us but strengthens us. We deserve to wake up every day feeling wonderful and disease free. Not dependent on medicine that causes more problems and is poisonous.


MY PREFERRED PLAN

**Step 1-** Dherb's 20 day Full Body Cleanse inclusive with proper recommended diet during Cleanse . Let it be noted here that you should stop with any and all other vitamins and supplements during the Cleanse period.

**Step2-**The next step, after completion of the 20 day Full Body Cleanse, is to begin the Essiac or 4 Herb Tea Regimen. Herbal Healer Academy and Dr. Marijah McCain are my recommended source as listed earlier. I personally use the 4

Herb Tea concentrate, but have also made the Essiac from herbs per original instructions. Either way this is a powerful and amazing daily supplement drink. It has the ability to help heal and cleanse and purify allowing your body to be more able to perform as it is supposed to. These four herbs work together to bring about maximum healing potential and in bringing the body back to a more balanced state of health thus allowing your immune system to work more proficiently. I also add Montana Yew Tips Extract into the tea once a day.

**Step 3-** At the same time I begin the 4 Herb Tea program I resume my Moringa Leaf Powder at 3 capsules once or twice a day. This to help build my body at the cellular level and supply it with much needed natural nutrients.

**Step 4-** I resume taking my Spirulina at 3 capsules once a day. I prefer a mix of Spirulina, Chlorella and Wheat Grass if available.

**Step5-** I continue the mostly raw and vegetarian diet and I continue juicing at least once a day. A note here; you can add the Spirulina and/ or the Moringa Leaf Powder in with the juiced vegetables.

**Step6-** I drink 8 glasses of filtered or alkaline water every day as to help my body to flush the toxins out. Obviously the best water to drink is the alkaline water, but filtered water will do. It is imperative that you stay hydrated and keep the ability to flush out the toxins ongoing to help bring about healing. A note once again concerning acidic and alkaline conditions. Finding a Naturopathic Doctor to work with especially concerning your pH is important if possible. Too acidic or too alkaline is both detrimental. So testing your pH level during any treatment needs to be consistent and ongoing.

This is pretty much my chosen plan for Cancer treatment. It is effective and the Essiac or 4 Herb Tea has been proven historically to be able to bring about a condition within your body that is conducive to healing. Make time for meditation or just relaxing and *"quieting your soul"* each day. Deep breathing each day will work wonders as a needed but overlooked activity in our lives. We so often shallow breathe if we are not active enough. Yes, we need activity and exercise. Even if you just walk every day, you need that exercise. Do something to get your heart and blood pumping and your lymph system moving.

I have written this book in the simplest terms I know how to. I do this because I believe everyone who seeks information and knowledge concerning any subject should be able to understand what they read and find. I hope you have been able to understand my writings and that you are encouraged to dig deeper and with an open mind to find what best suits you and what you are most comfortable with in dealing with Cancer. If nothing else I sincerely hope you realize that Cancer is not to be feared. That it can be cured or managed. There is life after Cancer and we all deserve a good and happy and healthy life.

# Chapter 9-Professionals Making a Difference

Here is a list of Doctors and others that are making a big difference in Cancer treatments and cures. Also, listed are some persons that are no longer with us but have made amazing contributions sometimes with the threat of jail and definitely ridiculed and ostracized by their own peers. There are many other pioneers past and present that have brought about healing Please feel free to find out more about each one and their work. God Bless……

Andreas Moritz
Dr. Marijah McCain
Julian Whitaker, M.D.
Rene Caisse R.N.
Jim Humble (jimhumble.org)
Otto Warburg
Dr. Stanislaw Burzynski
Dr. James Forsythe
Vernon "Vito" Johnston
Dr. Nicolas Gonzalez
Max Gerson and The Gerson Institute
Dherbs.com

# Source Information

**Sources:**

- www.essiacfacts.com this is an **extremely** informative website!!!
- http://newswithviews.com/ Howenstine/ james181.htm
- Knockout by Suzanne Somers
- www.phkillscancer.com
- www.nobelprize.org
- www.moringatoday.com/
- Vernon Johnston YouTube video on making baking soda solution. http://www.youtube.com/watch?v=Yl8Y8I_TsjI
- http://drsircus.com/
- www.wikapedia.org
- www.naturalnews.com
- www.fhcrc.org
- http://www.stopcancer.com/cancerwarrior3.htm
- www.cancer.gov
- www.NIH.gov
- http://www.cancer-treatment-tips.com/
- http://www.safesolutionsinc.com/Essiac_Tea.htm
- http://www.stopcancer.com/phhow_to_balance_your_body.htm
- "The Prime Cause and Prevention of Cancer" by Otto Warburg
- Lindau Lecture Writings by Otto Warburg
- http://alignlife.com/articles/toxicity/millions-falsely-treated-for-cancer-says-national-cancer-institute-report

# A Few Extra Research Sources

**A Few Extra Research Sources:**

- http://www.healthfreedom.info/
- https://www.facebook.com/eattobeat
- https://www.facebook.com/gersoninstitute
- https://www.facebook.com/essiacfacts
- https://www.facebook.com/pages/delicious-healthy-recipes/430642907050076

# Highly Recommended Reading List

Recommended Reading List:

The Bible

"You Can Heal Your Life" by Louise L. Hay

"Knockout" by Suzanne Summers

"Cancer Is Not a Disease-It's a Survival Mechanism" by Andreas Moritz

"The Master Key System" by Charles F Haanel

"I Want To Live Using Essiac" by Caroline Bennet

"Calling of An Angel" by Gary L Glum

"The Gerson Therapy" by Charlotte Gerson and D.P.M. Walker

# Other Books by the Author

**More Books by Daniel K Gartlan:**

"Poor Hannah"

"If It Was All About Me"

"Stones and Sticks: A Story About Bullying"

"14 Crazy Good Meatless Recipes for Eating Healthier"

"Princess Atnas of the North Pole and the Star of Wonder"

*__Coming in the late summer of 2016__*

*"South of Victory"*  *An American Civil War novel.*

# About the Author

Daniel Gartlan credits his mother for instilling in him a love of reading and writing. It is from this early influence that after 30 years in the business world, he has begun writing and publishing books from a diverse range of subjects. He likes to think of his writing style as simplistic as he strives to allow anyone reading his works to easily understand his subjects.

Daniel Gartlan resides with his wife in what he calls "Paradise" in the beautiful South Carolina Low-Country Islands of Beaufort, SC. Surrounded by his children and his 4 granddaughters he has much inspiration to brighten his days!